Lose Pounds Fast and Easy:

The Ultimate Weight Loss Solution and Low Calorie Recipe Book

By

Brittany Samons

Table of Contents

Lose Pounds Fast and Easy: The Ultimate Weight Loss
Solution and Low Calorie Recipe Book

By Brittany Samons

Introduction

If you think about indulging yourself what is the first idea that comes to your mind? Maybe eating a full bucket of popcorn while watching a movie or drinking that sweet soda which is in the fridge. Well let me explain to you the new meaning of "treating yourself": lose weight eat healthy food and exercise that is what I call treating yourself right. We will explore some tips on weight loss which bring benefits in this book. And everybody can easily follow them.

There's nothing that a good meal and exercise can't do for our bodies, there is nothing wrong in wanting to be slimmer but it is important to be healthy too.

Nothing New Under the Sun

For many years people have tried all kinds of diets: low carb diet, vegetarian diet, no grain diet, liquid diet, detox diet, paleolithic diet and the list goes on. The truth is that there is nothing new under the sun, there are a lot of diets that are trends right now they are the same diets the difference is the fancy names they have. There is no magic about a diet or another as every person is different the same happens with diets, not all diets are for all people, just find the one that works best for you, one that fits in your lifestyle and one that you embrace as part of your life but always remember the most important thing is to stay healthy.

Part 1. Weight Loss Tips

We are not going to delve in specific diets, here we will offer some easy and trusty tips about how to lose weight that you can incorporate in your everyday life.

1) Eat mindfully. Each time you eat try to be sitting at a table and having a plate and cutlery. This means you will be avoiding fast food (you are not going to eat a hamburger with a fork right!), by doing this it is probably you will be having a healthy dinner and avoid lots of unnecessary calories. It is proven people who eat mindfully consume fewer calories. Instead of using regular plates use salad plates, don't serve your drink in and oversized glasses instead use an eight-ounce glass. In a few days you will get used to it and you will eat less cutting down some pounds.

2) Exercise your mind. Having lack of willpower hold people from improving their lives, it is important to learn how to use it in our advantage. Every day we have choices to make: eat a slice of pizza or a vegetable frittata and here is where willpower needs to overcome and help us making the right decisions. Each time you have a craving try to remember healthy food is better, make the right choice!

3) Be realistic. Okay you want to lose weight, a lot, but what happened when it doesn't occur as fast as you expect? When you only drop 5 pounds? You get disappointed and go back to eat fried chicken. Not being realistic in which are our expectations is one of the biggest obstacles. You have to be conscious you are not going to be back on your school days weight. It is not the same 40 years than 20. Remember metabolism slows down with the age and it is our job to speed it. Having shed a pound or two each week is better than nothing. When you notice it you will have lost a lot of weight.

4) Take a look at your friends. If your friends like to have a drink every night after work then probably you will do it too, if your friends like to hang out for having oversized meals every Friday sure you will be eating an oversized meal too. Then the answer is choosing the right friends. Pick people with healthy habits and you will be doing healthier things. Instead of having beer and an oversized meal what about having a delicious salad and go for a walk. Have a "healthy night" each week, where you and your friends can cook some delicious food while having fun.

5) Checking your cart. Each time you go on a shopping trip to the supermarket check what it is in your cart. It should have in it some protein products, a few whole grains and lots of fruits and vegetables. Try to keep a grocery list with you, one that includes the ingredients for healthy breakfasts, lunches and dinners, this way you won't forget what you need to buy. Maybe you can get some snacks too (healthy snacks not a potato chips bag). Do not buy food that contains corn syrup or fructose. Look for a lower sugar version of that food (a light one) Buy sugar-free dressings and avoid partially hydrogenated foods.

6) Stop eating just because. Many people eat just because...because it is a birthday party, because what is a movie without cheesy nachos? If you really want to loss weight stop finding excuses to eat (remember the willpower issue?) There always is food at these events only eat when you are really hungry and don't overeat just because there are barbecue wings, pizza, hot dogs, ice cream, cake, soda, you have to try everything, no sir!

7) Eat fresh. Our lives are hectic these days, everybody is running to work, to pick up children at school, so there's no time for cooking but what if instead of grabbing frozen food at the supermarket you plan to go once a week to a farmer's market and buy fresh food then maybe you can pick a day and cook meals for all week. You will enjoy the trip and freed your body of chemicals. You can take your kids to the farmer's market so they could learn more about fresh vegetables and fruits, this way they will be adopting healthy habits too.

8) No night cravings. Once you had dinner, clean the kitchen and don't come back until next day in the morning. Eating late night increases the number of calories you eat. So no more sneaking in the middle of the night for snacking, this can save you 300 calories a day. Take your last dinner about 7:00 p.m. pour a glass of water and take it with you to your nightstand, if you feel like craving better take a sip.

9) Don't sabotage. People are used to sabotage themselves when dieting. We need to understand we are not going to get what we want or need from anybody else. It is important to learn how to validate us. You deserve to look good, to be good and to stay healthy so please don't eat that doughnut no matter if you are going to hit the gym for an hour. Love yourself, take a look at the mirror everyday and tell yourself how pretty you are. Feel good in your own skin and get confident.

10) Drink water. It is okay if you drink an orange juice in the morning but the rest of the day stick to water. Do you know that you can consume an extra 245 calories by drinking a soda? That's a lot! Besides soda don't quench your thirst. Water is good for the body, for the skin, for the brain, and guess what? It is a lot cheaper than soda o sweetened drinks.

11) Do not choose white. People are so used to eat white bread and white rice. White flour contains large amounts of carbohydrates and added sugar, imagine what this will do to your body, you can still eat bread and rice choose whole grain breads and brown rice. White flours are too processed, that is why Paleo Diet proposes to get rid of them. Paleolithic people didn't eat processed foods, only whole grain flours.

12) Black coffee please. Coffee shops have evolved and offer a wide variety of coffee drinks. Imagine how many more calories are you drinking thanks to whole milk, syrup, whipped cream and chocolate chips. If you have one of those fancy coffees everyday get for sure your weight will go to the sky! Next time you grab a coffee ask for a black one with skim milk. It will be cheaper and healthier. Of course you can have one of those sugary drinks once a week.

13) If you can't resist choose the correct snack. A boiled egg maybe with a teaspoon of mayonnaise it's a good snack with low calories and protein. Dark chocolate is another good choice of a healthy snack (just a piece not the complete bar!) If you are a yogurt fan guess what? It is good too especially Greek yogurt and low fat yogurt. All kinds of nuts help keep your hunger in control, prepare your own trail mix with dried fruit, raisins, nuts and seeds.

14) Set Goals. It is important to establish a goal when losing weight; it is not just about lost weight, how are you going to achieve it? Goals must be specific, realistic and timely, this way it would be easier to achieve them. For example if you think about exercising it is a goal but if you say I will go to the gym everyday and exercise for 30 minutes is a precise goal. Or if you are thinking about taking ballroom classes every day probably you won't do it, but if you try it 2 days a week is a good beginning.

15) Don't spend all day on a chair. Many people spend a significant timespan sitting behind a desk while working. If it is your case try to move as much as you can, remain standing during a call, walk to the cafeteria instead of order in, take the stairs and avoid the elevator, if it is possible walk to work, every step counts! It would be a good idea to carry a pedometer with you and set a goal for each day maybe 500 more steps than the day before. It is a simple equation more steps less weight.

You can compete with your co-workers who set the walking record!

16) Cleaning Time. It is a great exercise to make some house chores. Remember the idea is being active. Hand wash dishes instead of using the dishwasher, go upstairs to pick up laundry, wash your car, sweep is great too for burning calories!

Maybe this doesn't sound very appealing but you will have to it so what about listening your favorite music while cleaning?

17) Gardening. You can rake leaves from your garden once a week, take care of your plants and trees, take out weed and remove the ground, this way you are keeping your garden nice while cutting down some fat. In winter time remove snow from your front door, maybe you can help your neighbors.

18) Learn to relax. I don't think it is possible to be without stress in our lives. Stress can be a good source in gaining weight, if you handle stress by eating a candy bar now and a brownie later, weight will go on and on. If work is stressing you out take a break, walk for ten minutes instead of eating a chocolate muffin. Take some yoga classes, once a month indulges you with a visit to the spa.

19) Listen to your body. We are used to eat because we are bored, nervous, frustrated, it is just a bad habit, sometimes we actually forget how does being hungry feels. If you eat anything is near you probably it is not hunger just a craving. Learn to listening your body, when your stomach mumbles it will probably means you are hungry, not when your brain is saying eat the cookie.

20) Keep a diary. Studies have shown that people who keep a record of their meals eat less food, so what are you waiting for? Write down what you eat every week and be careful with weekends; people consume extra calories on weekends. Cut out calories by avoiding salad dressings, soda and unhealthy snacks.

21) No more T.V. shows Try to reduce the number of hours you spend in front of the TV. It is true that people eat more while watching TV. Instead of eating a bag of microwave popcorn and watch a show, take your dog out for a walk, both of you will benefit.

22) Give away your clothes. When you notice you are losing weight get rid of those big clothes, the idea of buying a new wardrobe is a great incentive to keep the right weight, nobody wants to go back to those "fatty clothes". It also is a good charity to give things to people who need them.

Part 2. Low Calorie Recipes

Often when people are following a diet they made up many excuses to skip their healthy meals, it is boring, it's always the same, it's not delicious.

Below we are offering some easy, delicious and healthy recipes you can try without making up excuses.

Honey and Mustard Pork Chops

188 calories. 4 servings

Ingredients

- 4 pork chops (1 pound approximately)

- 1/8 teaspoon of ground black pepper

- 3 tablespoons of soy sauce

- 1 tablespoon of honey

- 1 tablespoon of Dijon mustard

- 1 teaspoon of garlic, minced

Step 1 First spray a large saucepan with oil, medium-high heat. Sprinkle both sides of the chops with pepper and place them on the saucepan. Cook for about 3 or 4 minutes or until chops are slightly crispy.

Step 2 Turn the chops and cook for 2 or 3 more minutes until they are slightly pink in the center. Set aside and keep warm.

Step 3 Add the rest of the ingredients to the saucepan. Cook at mid-high heat for about a minute or until the mix boil. Stirring often.

Step 4 Serve the pork chops and pour honey and mustard sauce on them.

202 calories, 4 servings

Ingredients

- 4 boneless and skinless chicken breasts

- 1/2 cup of bread crumbs (preferably chose whole grain bread)

- 1/2 teaspoon of garlic salt

- 1 teaspoon of pepper

- 1 teaspoon of lemon zest

- 1/4 cup or lemon juice

- 2 tablespoons of canola oil

Step 1 First preheat the oven at 375°F. Spray an oven tray with oil.

Step 2 Mix in a Ziploc bag the breadcrumbs, garlic salt, pepper and lemon zest.

Steps 3 In other Ziploc bag mix the lemon juice with the oil.

Step 4 Add chicken breasts into the bag with the lemon juice and shake it, take them out and place them in the other bag. Shake until they get covered with the mix.

Step 5 Place the chicken in the oven tray, sprinkle the rest of the breadcrumbs mixture on top. Cook for 20 to 25 minutes or until the chicken is no pink on the inside.

You can serve with a green lettuce or spinach salad or with some vegetables you like.

222 calories, 6 servings

Ingredients

- 1 pound of ground beef lean meat

- 1/2 teaspoon of salt

- 1/4 teaspoon of garlic powder

- 2 cups of low sodium beef broth
- 1 can (14.5 oz) tomatoes, diced

- 2 cups of mixed vegetables (better if they are fresh)

- 1-1/2 cups of brown rice, uncooked

Step 1 First in a skillet cook the meat with salt and garlic powder, mid-high heat, until meat is in crumbs and no more pink color.

Step 2 Add the rest of the ingredients into the skillet, stir to mix together.

Step 3 Lei it boil and reduce heat to mid-low. Cook for about 5 minutes or until rice gets tender. Instead of a skillet you can use a Dutch oven.

306 calories, 4 servings

Ingredients

- 1/3 cup of orange ginger stir fry marinade sauce

- 1 can (11oz) of tangerines, drained (reserve juice)

- 1 tablespoon of honey

- 1 tablespoon of canola oil

- 1 pound of boneless and skinless chicken breasts cut in strips.

- 1 package (6 oz) of baby spinach leaves.

- 1/4 cup of almonds

Step 1 In a small bowl mix the stir-fry sauce with the tangerine juice you reserved and the honey. Set aside.

Step 2 Heat oil in a large pan, medium-high heat. Add the chicken and cook until the chicken is well cooked, stir occasionally.

Step 3 Add the sauce mix and wait until it boils. Cook for about 2 or 3 minutes or until the mix simmer slightly. Let it cool.

Step 4 Divide the spinach in four plates for serving. Cover with the chicken and the tangerines. Garnish with a few almonds.

118 calories, 4 servings

Ingredients

- 2 cans (5 oz each) of natural tuna, drained

- 1/2 cup of carrots chopped

-1/4 cup radish chop in quarters

- 1/4 cup green onion sliced

- 1/4 cup sweet and sour souce

- 2 teaspoons of soy sauce

- 8 large lettuce leaves

Step 1 In a medium size bowl mix the tuna with the carrots, radishes, green onions and both sauces.

Step 2 Place a lettuce leaf on a plate, put a spoonful of the tuna mix and wrap forming a roll. Serve.

If you like something crunchy you can add peanuts or nuts over each roll.

Spinach Nut Italian Penne

387 calories, 4 servings

Ingredients

- 2 cups low sodium vegetable broth

- 1 can (14.5) tomatoes with basil, garlic and oregano

- 2 cups of penne pasta, uncooked

- 2 tablespoons of butter

- 1 tablespoon of olive oil

- 1 package (6 oz) baby spinach leaves

- 1/3 cup chopped nuts

- 1/2-cup Parmesan cheese grated

Step 1 First in a large saucepan mix the broth with the tomatoes, penne and butter. High heat until boil, stirring occasionally. Cover the saucepan, low heat and cook during 15 minutes or until pasta is tender. Stirring.

Step 2 Next add the spinach leaves and stir. Before serving, sprinkle nuts and the cheese over the top.

380 calories, 4 servings

Ingredients

- 4 large whole grain flour tortillas

- 1/2 cup of peanut butter

- 6 tablespoons of granola or trail mix of your preference

- 1 red apple peeled

Step 1 Spread two spoonful of peanut butter on each tortilla, put some granola or trail mix on it.

Step 2 Next cut the apple in quarters, rid the seeds and cut in smaller pieces. Place them on each tortilla.

Step 3 Begin to roll each tortilla and wrap both ends to enclose like a burrito.

212 calories, 4 servings

Ingredients

- 4 large potatoes to bake

- 1/4 cup of sour cream low fat

- 1 tablespoon of butter

- 1 teaspoon of salt

- 1/8 teaspoon ground black pepper

- 1 cup egg substitute (Egg Beaters)

- 2 cup of broccoli florets cooked and drained

Step 1 Wrap in plastic foil each potato individually and place them on a microwaveable plate. Cook during 5 minutes at high temperature. Turn potatoes and then cook for 4 more minutes or until smooth.

Step 2 Once potatoes are cool cut them in halves. Remove the inner part and leave the skin. Place potatoes on a medium plate.

Step 3 In a bowl add sour cream, butter salt and pepper, use an immersion blender at slow speed until puree or desired consistency.

Step 4 Spray oil in a medium pan and low heat. Add the eggbeaters and cook without stirring until the bottom begins to settle.

Step 5 Add broccoli florets and stir slowly.

Step 6 Next add the eggs to the potato puree and move. Pour the mix into the potatoes shell and microwave for about 4 minutes at high temperature or until they are hot.

You can sprinkle some lemon juice on top. This could be a great lunch or dinner.

245 calories, 8 servings

Ingredients

- 1 cup of brown beans, drained

- 1 cup of fresh carrots finely chopped

- 1 can (15 oz) of Sloppy Joe Sauce

- 4 cups of water

- 1 tablespoon of brown sugar

- 8 hamburger buns (preferably choose whole grain bread)

Step 1 First in a large pot mix beans and water. Cover with a lid and mid-heat until boil.

Step 2 Once the beans are boiling add the chopped carrots. Low temperature to mid-low and cook for 20 minutes or until beans are tender. Drain.

Step 3 Next add the brown sugar and Sloppy Joe sauce, cook for 5 minutes stir often.

Step 4 Place the beans on the buns and serve immediately.

Serve these burgers with lettuce leaves.

278 calories, 6 servings

Ingredients

- 1/2 cup of low fat sour cream

- 1 can (10 0z) tomatoes diced and drained

- 1/2 cup lime juice

- fresh cilantro finely chopped

- 3 cups of cabbage mix (three colors)

- 1-1/2 pounds of tilapia fillets (no frozen)

- 1/2 teaspoon of salt

- 1 tablespoon of canola oil

- 12 corn tortillas

Step 1 In a small bowl mix sour cream, water from tomatoes until a sauce is made. Set aside.

Step 2 In other medium bowl combine tomatoes and cabbage mix. Set aside.

Step 3 Next season the tilapia fillets with salt. Heat the oil in a large pan mid-high temperature. Place the fillets and cook for 3 or 4 minutes each side, or until is tender and well cooked.

Step 4 Divide fish in 12 pieces and toss them in each tortilla. Cover with 1/4 cup of cabbage salad and 1 tablespoon of sauce. Fold the tortillas and serve immediately.

367 calories, 4 servings

Ingredients

- 8 oz. dry spaghetti, uncooked

- 1-cup peas (preferably choose fresh peas)

- 1/2 cup of egg beaters

- 1/2 cup of cream (use low fat)

- 1/2 cup of milk (skim milk can be used)

- 1/4 cup parmesan cheese, grated

- 1/4 teaspoon ground black pepper

- 1/3 cup (6 oz) of turkey pepperoni cut in quarters

Step 1 First cook spaghetti as package cooking directions. Two minutes before spaghetti is ready add the peas.

Step 2 Meanwhile in a glass microwaveable bowl place the eggs, milk, cream, the cheese and the pepper. Stir to mix together all the ingredients.

Step 3 Cook in the microwave for 30 seconds at high temperature. Stir again until is all blended.

Step 4 Drain spaghetti and peas and get them back in the pot. Add the turkey pepperoni and slowly add the eggs mix, stirring. Serve immediately.

You can replace turkey pepperoni for turkey bacon

Caramel Spice Eggnog

111 calories, 8 servings

Ingredients

- 4 cups (3,25 oz each) caramel and butterscotch pudding

- 1-cup egg beaters

- 1/2 teaspoon of pumpkin pie spices

- 1 can (12 oz) low fat evaporate milk

- 2 tablespoon of brown sugar

- 1/2 teaspoon of rum

- Dairy Whipped Topping (optional)

Step 1 First beat the pudding, the egg beaters and spices in a large bowl until everything is well blended.

Step 2 Add the milk, brown sugar and rum, stir together.

Step 3 Serve immediately. Cover with whipped topping if you like it.

Being on a diet doesn't mean you can't indulge yourself with some low calorie desserts.

Conclusion

It doesn't matter what diet you choose what really matters is to set smart goals and have a healthy life, weight loss is important to achieve this. We have mentioned some fabulous tips that are very easy to put on practice even if your schedule is a little tight. Some of them are daily tasks that you are avoiding or forgetting about.

The recipes in this article are only a few examples of healthy food, easy to prepare in a short period of time and it is also delicious. You can research for more recipes and try cooking more often instead of buying prepared food. Do not forget to eat fresh!

I want to personally thank you for reading my book. I hope you found information in this book useful and I would be very grateful if you could leave your honest review about this book. I certainly want to thank you in advance for doing this.

9 781633 832718